I dedicate this book
to my hero, **Guy Bryant.**
He has brought nothing but
love and joy into my life.

Introduction

Does your child have a friend, family member, or classmate who has poop or pee accidents? Would you like your child or children to understand more about bowel or bladder accidents? Are you looking for an engaging way to start a dialogue about these problems? I wrote this book to help solve these challenges.

P is for Poop and Pee Accidents is a children's picture book in an ABC format. This book teaches common issues in people with these kinds of accidents with delightful illustrations. A child who has accidents narrates this book from his (or her) point of view.

As with my previous books, I deliberately focused on a child with more significant bowel and bladder problems. Some children may have only bladder accidents. Some children never have bladder accidents and jump right to bowel accidents. The child in this book sees a doctor who provides a treatment plan to address his/her issues. I cannot stress enough that a trained professional should address your child's bowel and bladder problems. This book should only prepare you for the types of treatment that a medical professional might recommend.

I hope *P is for Poop and Pee Accidents* provides an entertaining way to start a simple educational discussion about managing bowel and bladder difficulties. I invite you to read this story interactively with your child. Encourage discussions of how you or people you love might be like the child in this book. You might compare and contrast how the child in this book is similar or different from someone you know with bowel or bladder management difficulties. This book provides essential opportunities to discuss how to be a friend to a child who experiences these kinds of problems.

As a pediatric physical therapist, I work with children who have accidents. Unfortunately, others often misunderstand the actions and behaviors of people who experience such difficulties. As a result, people can be very unkind to children with these kinds of accidents. I believe knowledge helps break down barriers and encourages kindness and patience. Assisting children to understand poop and pee accidents at a young age is powerful. I hope this book provides knowledge and empowerment for your child.

P is for Poop and Pee Accidents

A Child's View

Published by **Gotcha Apps, LLC**
1904 ½ Williams St.
Valdosta, GA 31602

This book provides general information on bowel and bladder difficulties
and management. It should not be relied upon as recommending or
promoting any specific diagnosis or method of treatment.
It is not intended as a substitute for medical advice or direct
diagnosis and treatment of encopresis or enuresis by
a qualified physician or therapist.

Readers who have questions about bowel and bladder management
or its treatment should consult with a physician, counselor,
or other qualified health care professional.

ISBN:978-1-7365307-1-9

Cover art and interior artwork by **Ikos Ronzkie**

Text by **Amy E. Sturkey, PT**

P is for Poop and Pee Accidents

written by
Amy E. Sturkey, PT

illustrated by
Ikos Ronzkie

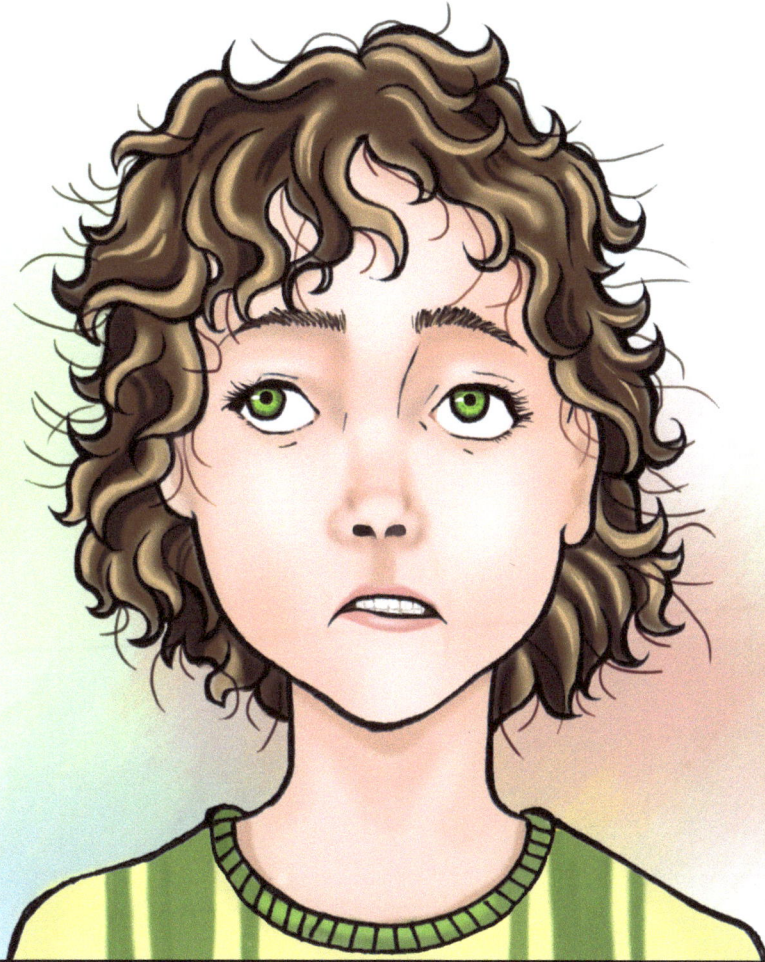

A is for an Accident--just a
teeny tiny little one at night.
I was already potty trained during the day.
I could stay dry at night with no problem.
So I could not believe it when I woke one
morning and found that I had wet the bed!
Oh no! Who knew this would be the
beginning of a huge problem?

B is for Bedwetting.
Bedwetting became a once
every few days problem and
then an every night problem.
My belly started to hurt
almost every day.

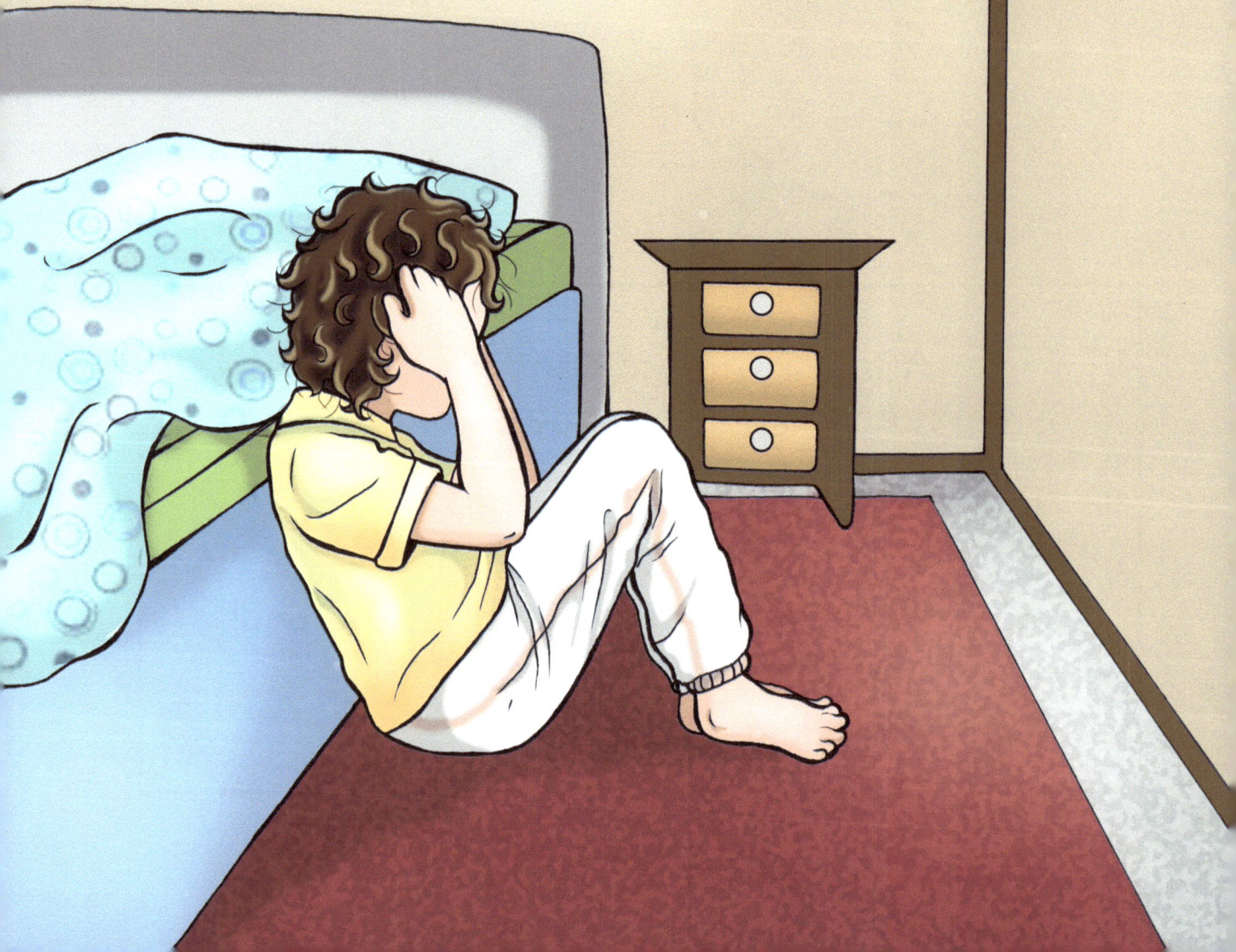

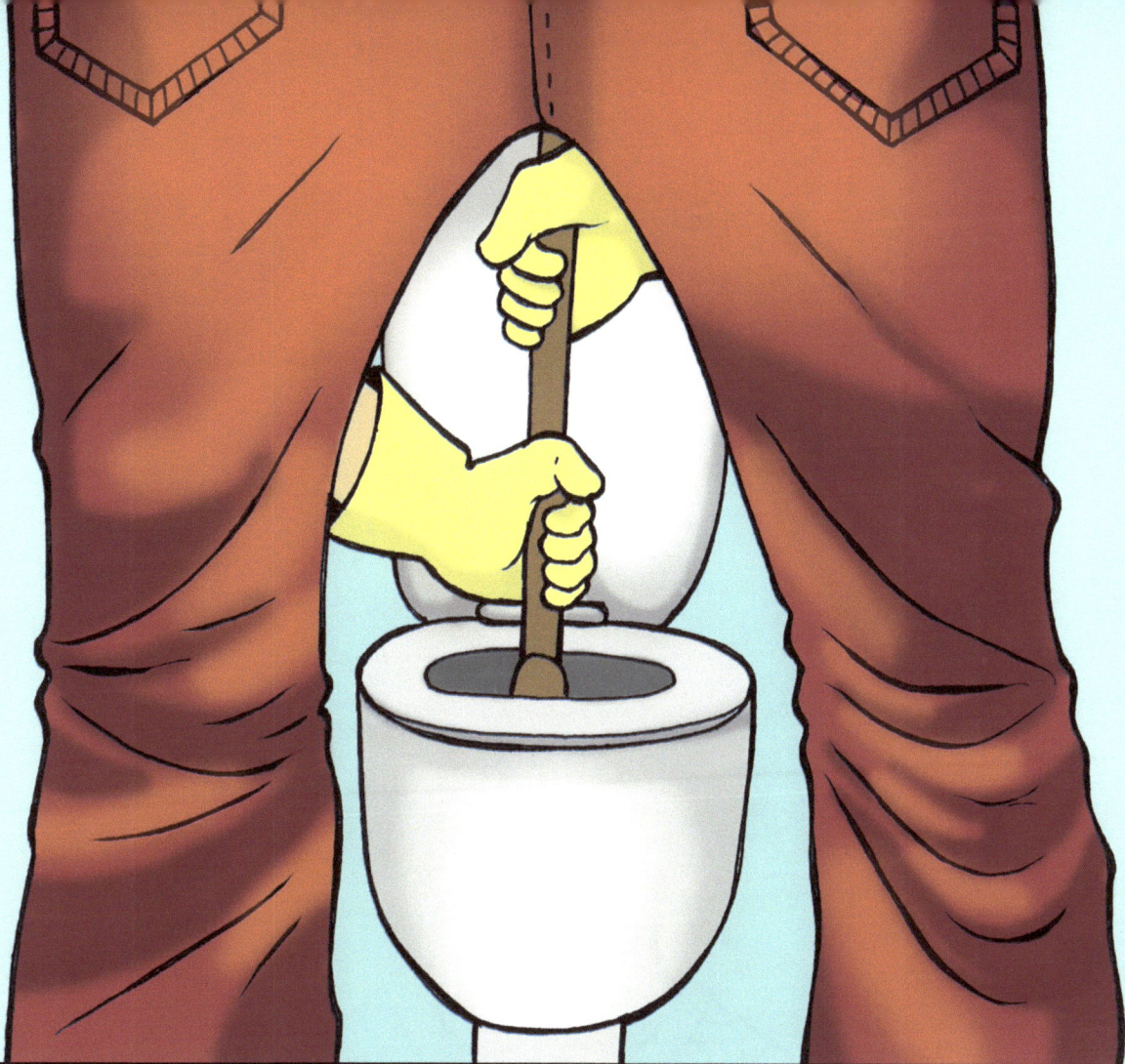

C is for Clogging the toilet.
I can't believe that came out of my bottom!
That is too big! Mom said I must be constipated.
She explained constipation is when you don't poop
often enough or get all the poop out in one sitting.
The poop is difficult to squeeze out. It is dry and hard.
Most people say you are constipated if you have less
than three poops a week for two weeks. That's true,
but you can also be constipated if you poop too many
times a day. You might have a big hard poop inside that
is blocking all the poop from coming out at once.

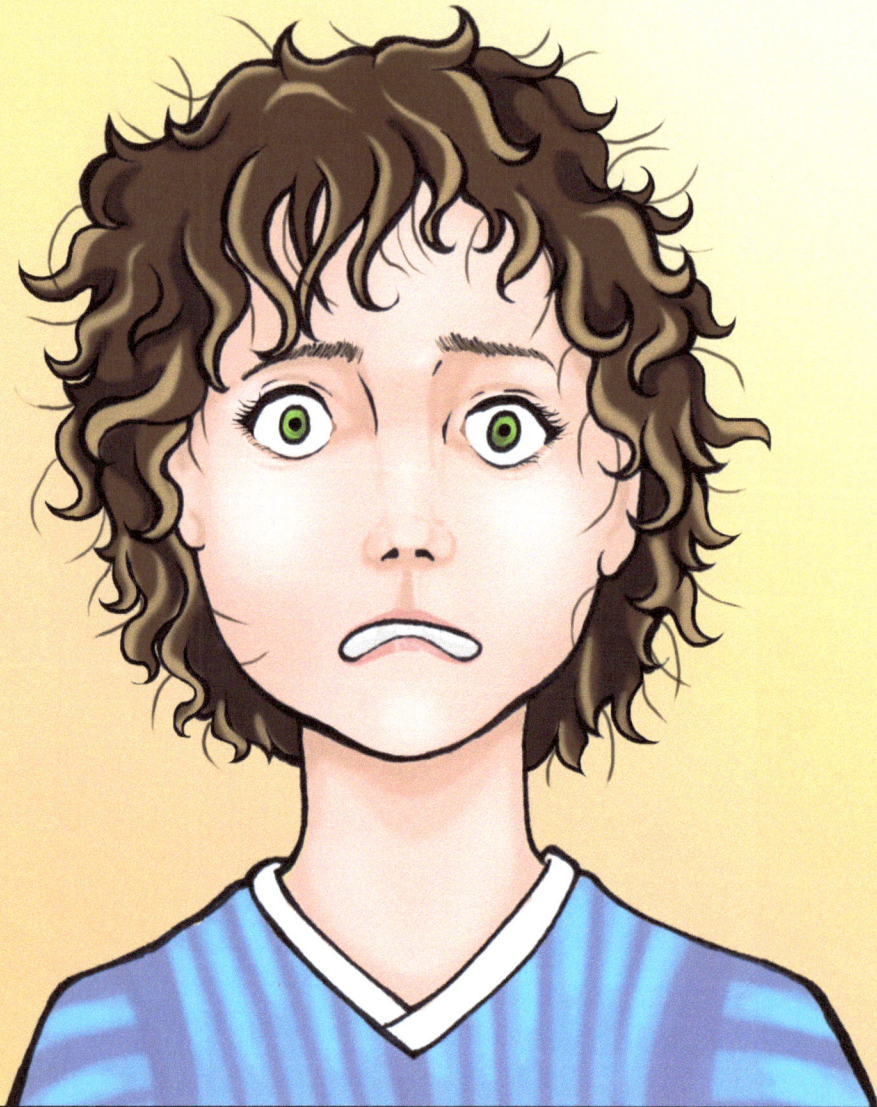

D is for Daytime pee accidents.
That is what happened next.
Can you believe it? Yes, I just peed.
I leaked pee in my underwear!
What is going on?

E is for Embarrassment.
How could it get any worse? Eeek! My Dad says
every day I need to poop! But, I do not feel like
I need to poop. When I do--no matter how much
I strain, push, and make faces, I just can't poop.
I only poop once or twice a week.

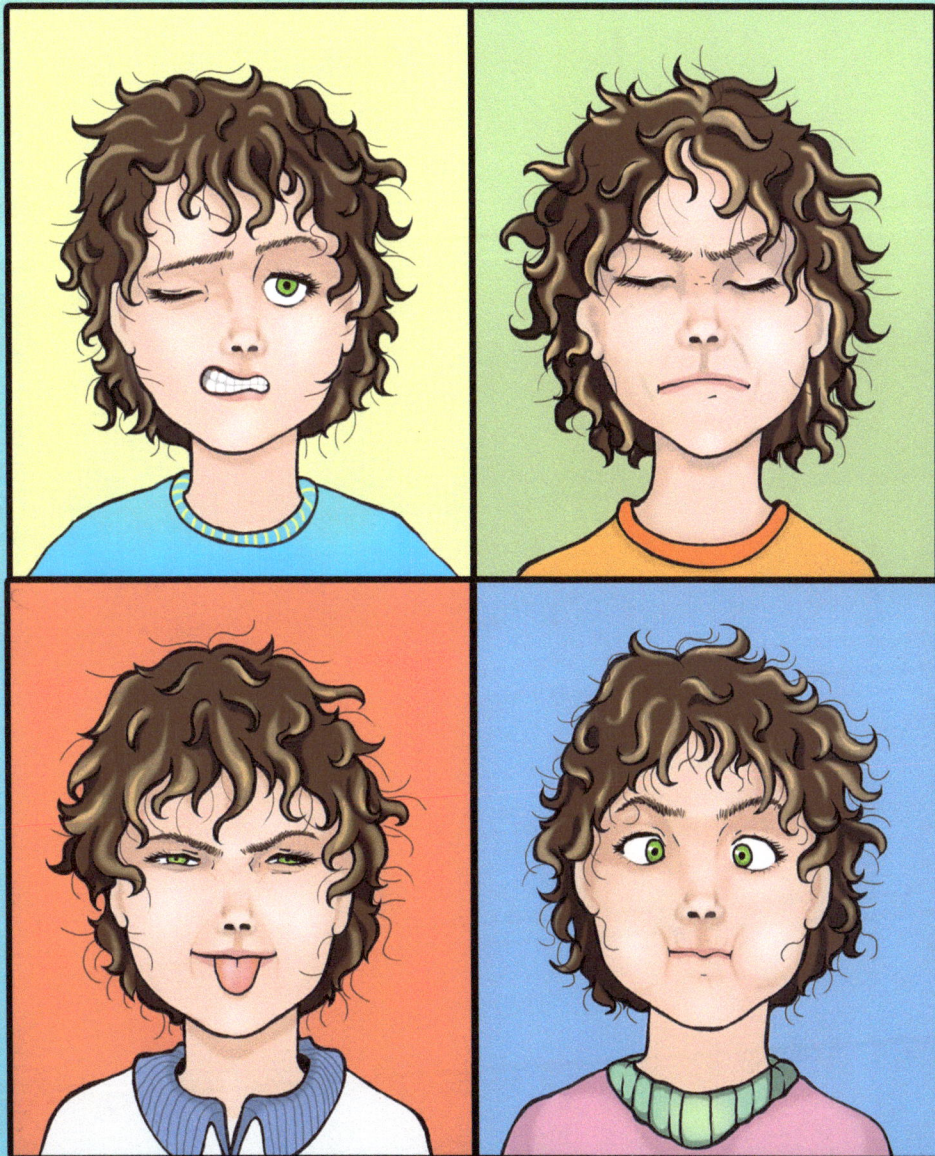

F is for Falling out.
This is the day the poop hit the fan--poop
started oozing out onto my underwear.
What!?! Why can't I feel it? Why can't I smell it?
Everyone else can. And boy, do they let me know!
Later on, little poop pellets just fell out on
their own. How am I going to make it
through this school year?

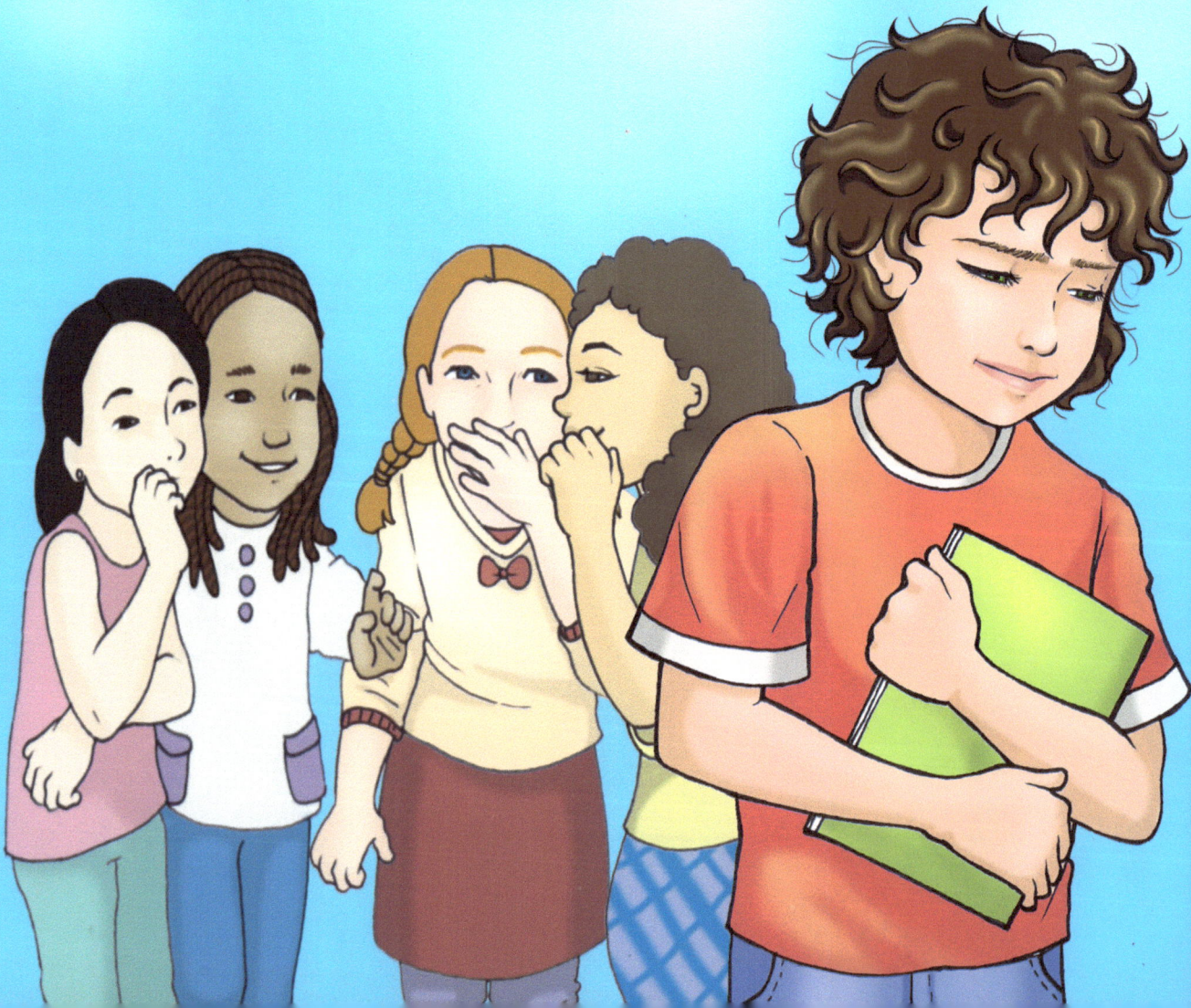

G is for a Great big problem.
I need to have extra clothes at school.
I am bullied by the mean kids and teased by the
nice kids--even Emma. I don't want to ask the teacher
to go to the bathroom. I don't want to go to the
bathroom at school with the other kids around.
I don't want to go to school at all. Good golly,
this can't get any worse.

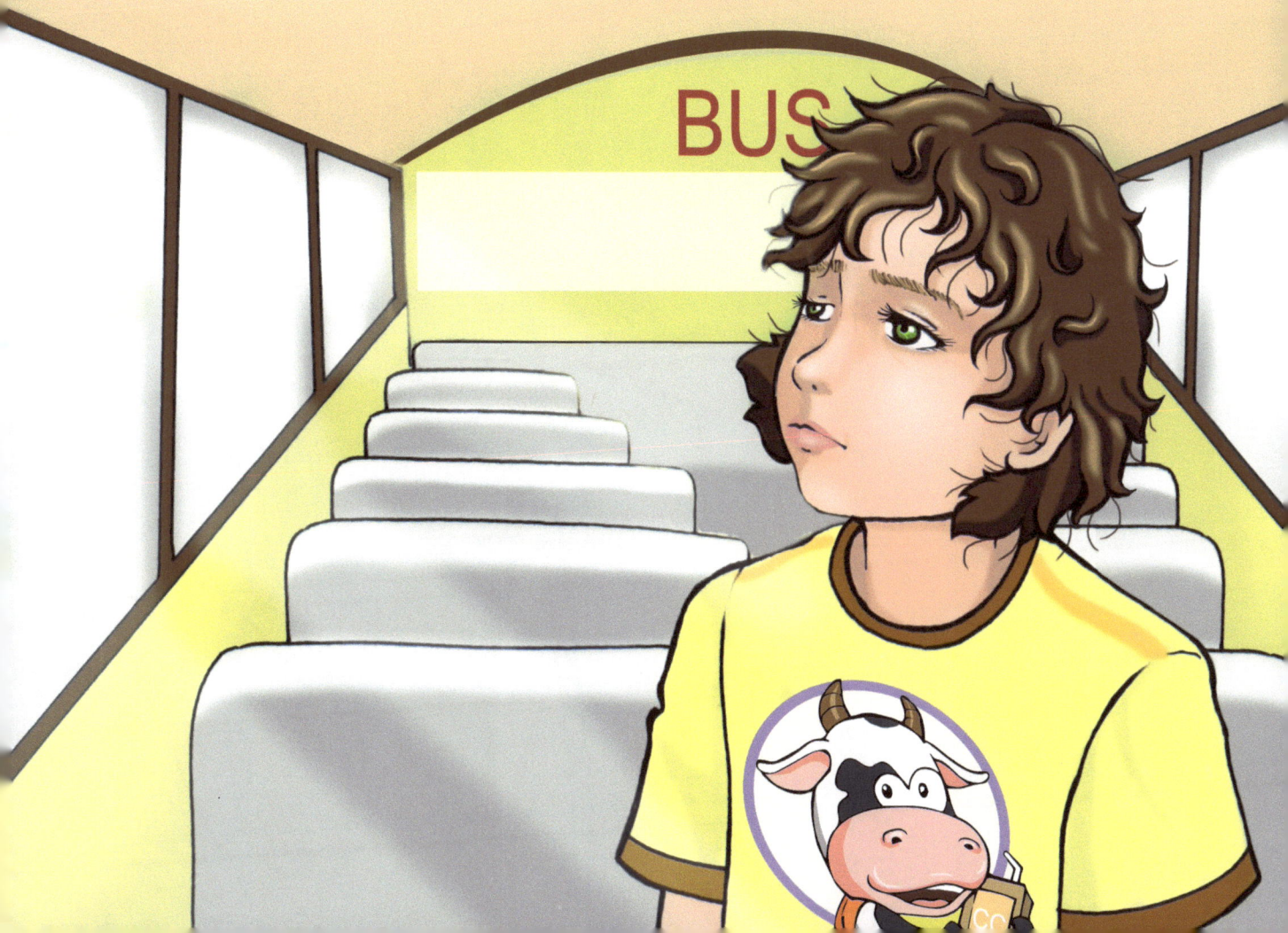

H is for Help.
This is when my parents took me to
a doctor who explained this wasn't my fault.
So we made a plan to help me.

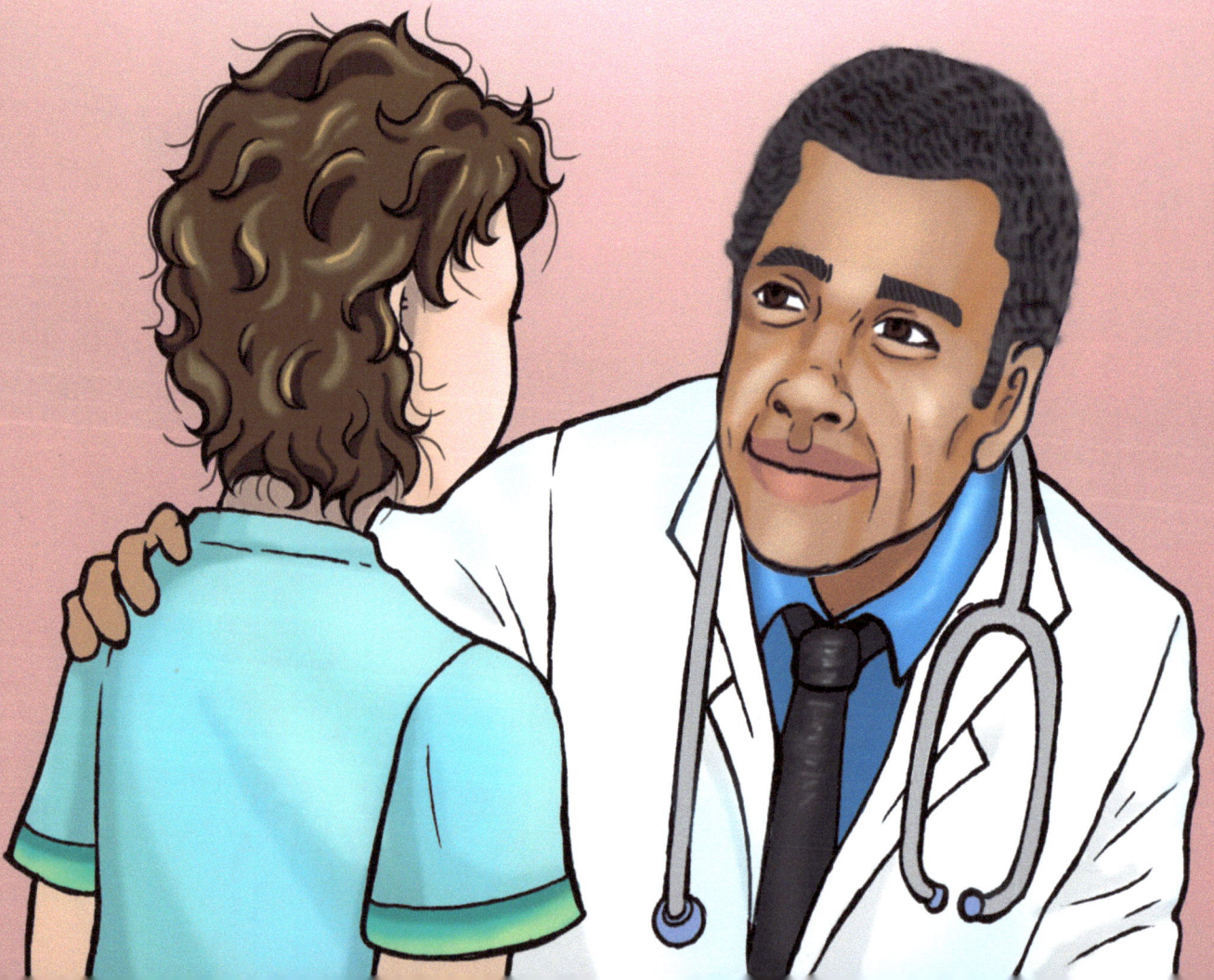

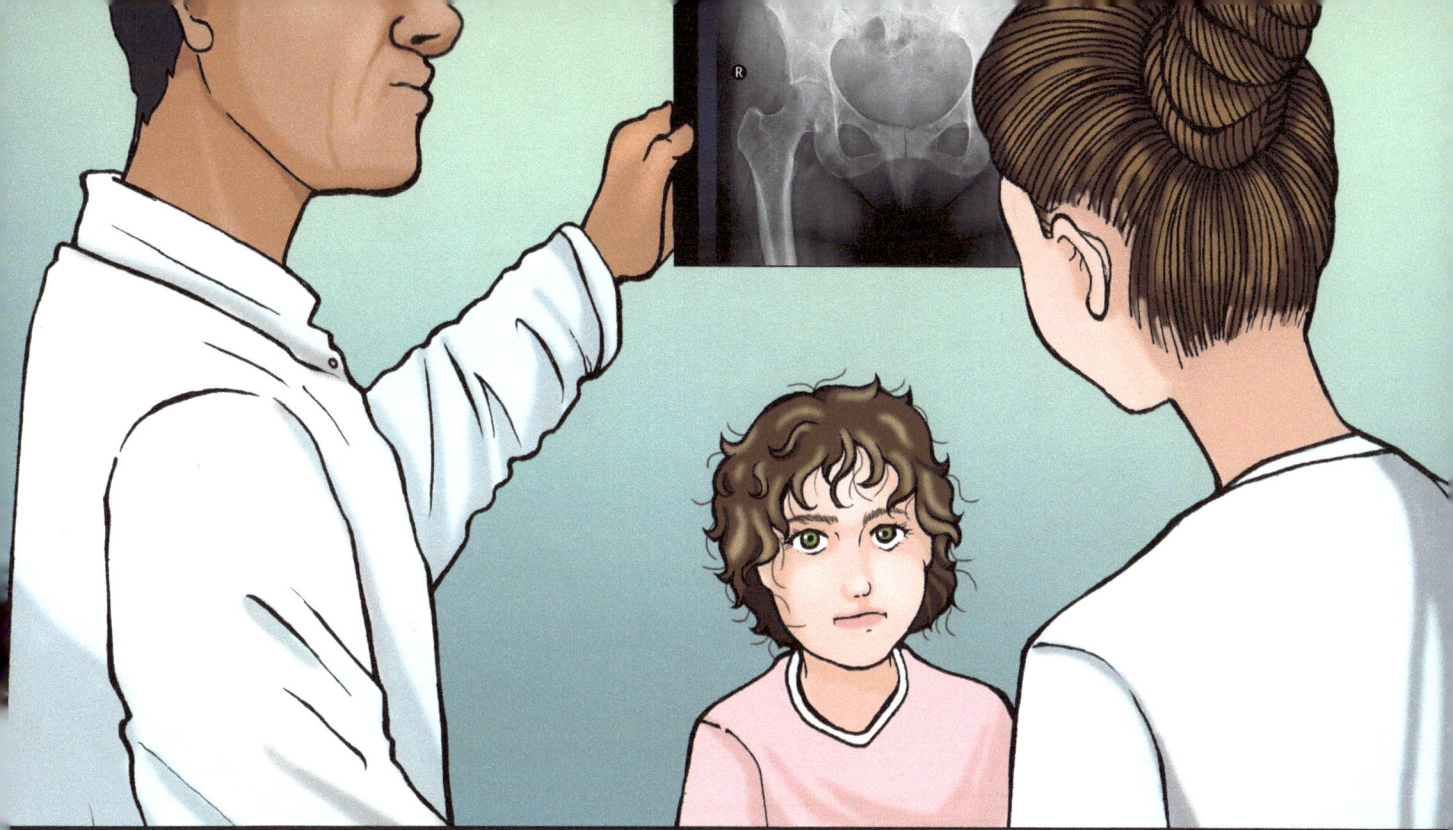

I is for I didn't know.

I had no idea that a bunch of poop blocked up inside of me caused all my problems. I had an X-ray that showed the truth. My poops were so backed up that only watery poop, poop pellets, or toilet cloggers were getting through. The poop was pressing on my bladder and nerves, causing pee hiccups that I couldn't control. The doctor said almost 90% of the time, backed-up poop is the problem for kids with poop or pee accidents.

J is for Just.

The doctor said that just taking laxatives or stool softeners, changing the food I eat, going to the bathroom on a schedule, and drinking more water will probably **NOT** be enough to fix my problem. Instead, he explained that the research says daily enemas are the best answer to getting that poop out and keeping it from backing up again. An enema is a liquid that is placed in my rectum to help get the poop out. The rectum is the last place poop is kept before it comes out of my body.

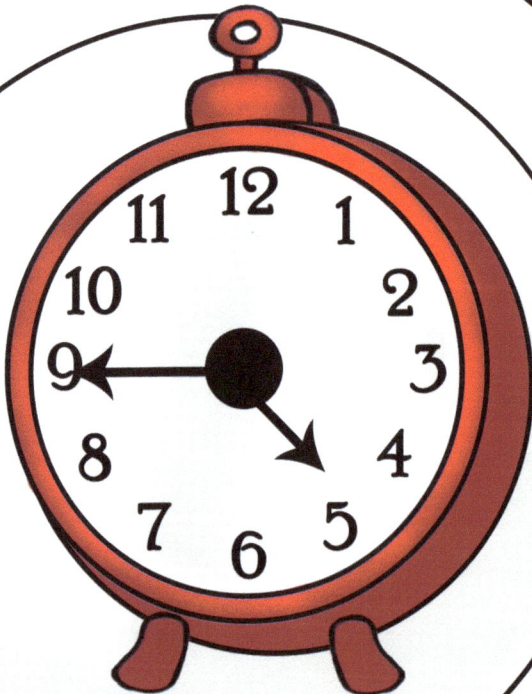

Life-Saving Plan

1. Eat Real Food
2. Toileting Schedule
3. Drink more water
4. Exercise
5. Daily Enema

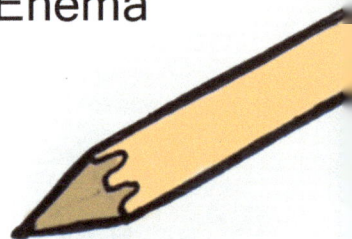

K is for Keep.

I must really try hard to keep the poop from bunching up inside me and stretching out my rectum. This process takes at least three months! Constant constipation has completely overstretched my rectum, making it a pond instead of a dirt road. I have to help it get back down to normal size. Then I will know when I need to go poop. When my bladder is no longer smooshed and hiccupping, I won't have pee accidents anymore. Then, I will make it to the bathroom in plenty of time.

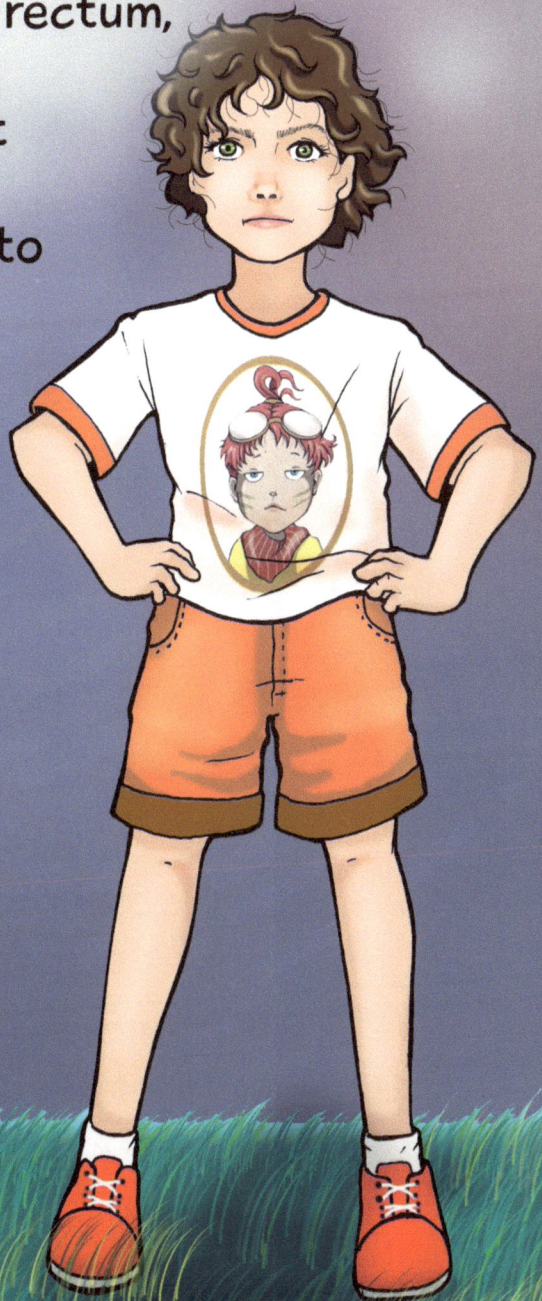

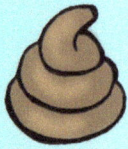

soft serve ice cream

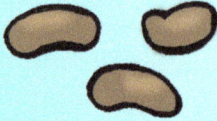

soft sausages

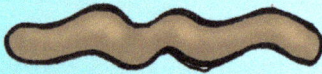

smooth snakes

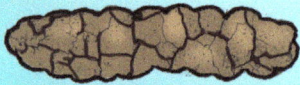

thick lumpy cracked sausages

crowded grapes

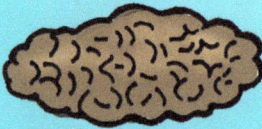

corn on the cob

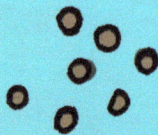

little hard balls

L is for Look.

I have to look at my poops to see how I am doing. Poops formed like soft serve ice cream, soft sausages, or smooth snakes are great. I have a problem if my poops are thick lumpy cracked sausage, long tough logs, crowded grapes, corn on the cob, or little hard balls.

M is for Most likely.

I am most likely to poop
15 to 30 minutes after I eat.
I always sit on the toilet after
getting up in the morning, after
each meal, and before bedtime.
I sit on the toilet for 3 to 10
minutes at a time. If I do poop,
I stay 1-2 minutes longer,
just to make sure more
isn't coming.

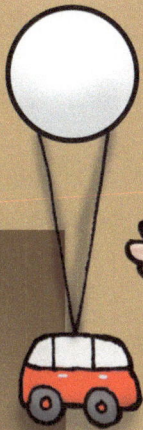

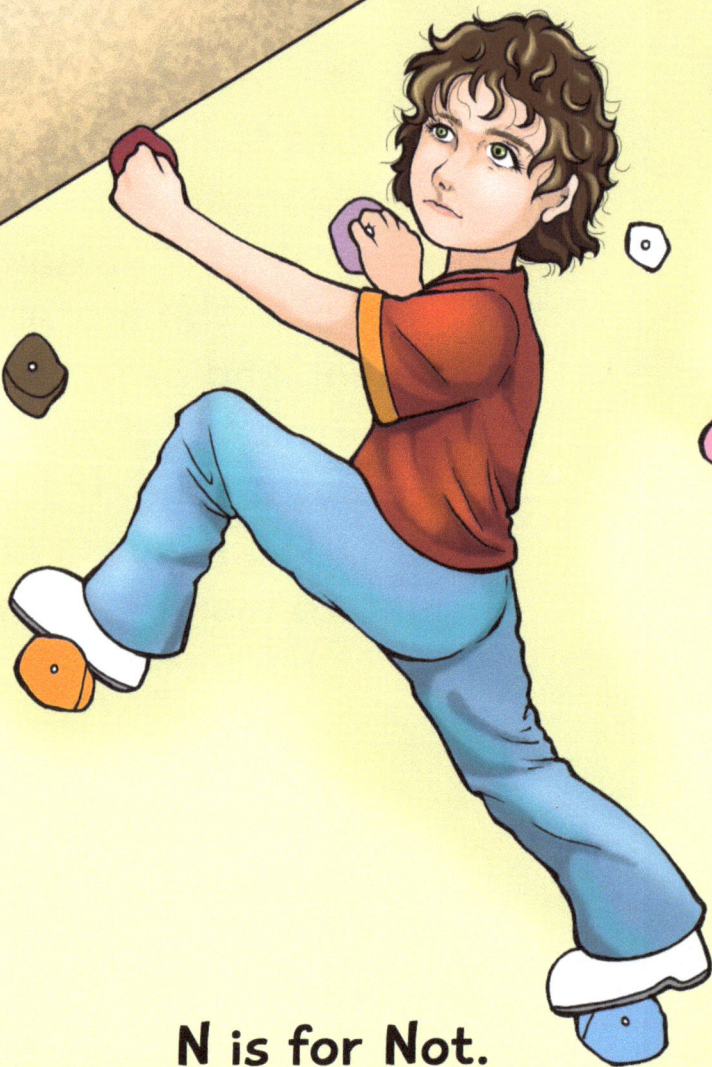

N is for Not.
I had to learn not to ignore my urges
or hold my poop. Until my poops get down
to normal size, my poops might be uncomfortable.
Sometimes having to poop might be inconvenient.
I may have to leave something fun or ask the
teacher if I can go to the bathroom.
Holding my poop was part
of my problem.

O is for Obviously.

Obviously, my days of hiding my underwear with poop on them are over. My Mom and Dad are helping me. The teacher is helping, too. I have a secret hand signal to let my teacher know when I need to go to the bathroom. She understands now how important it is. In addition, I can change clothes in a private restroom if I need.

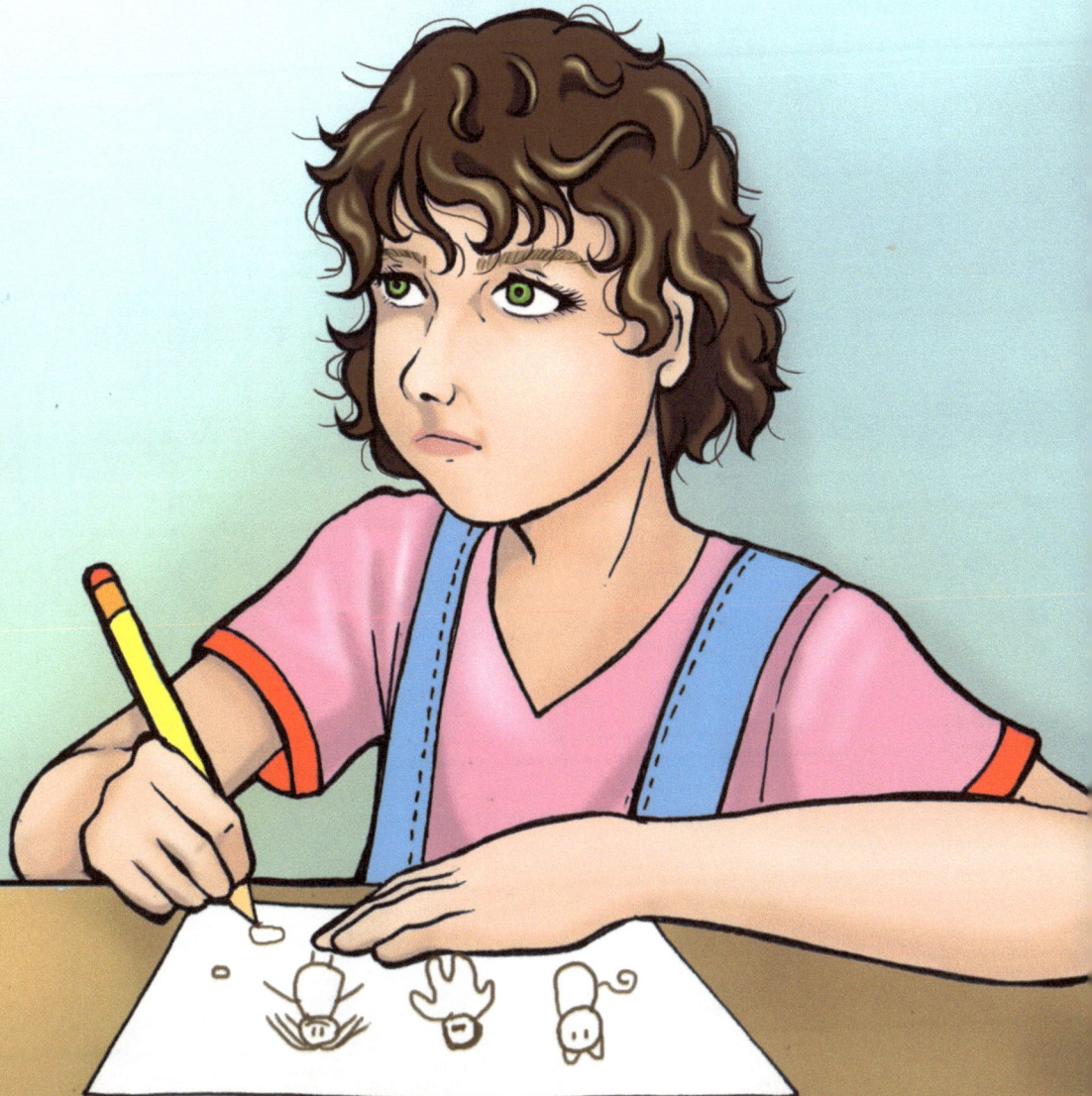

P is for Potty Posture.

I am more likely to poop and pee more completely if I sit on a toilet with my knees higher than my hips. So I put my feet on a tall stool. I lean forward with my back straight, with my elbows on my knees to help me relax so my poop comes out more easily.

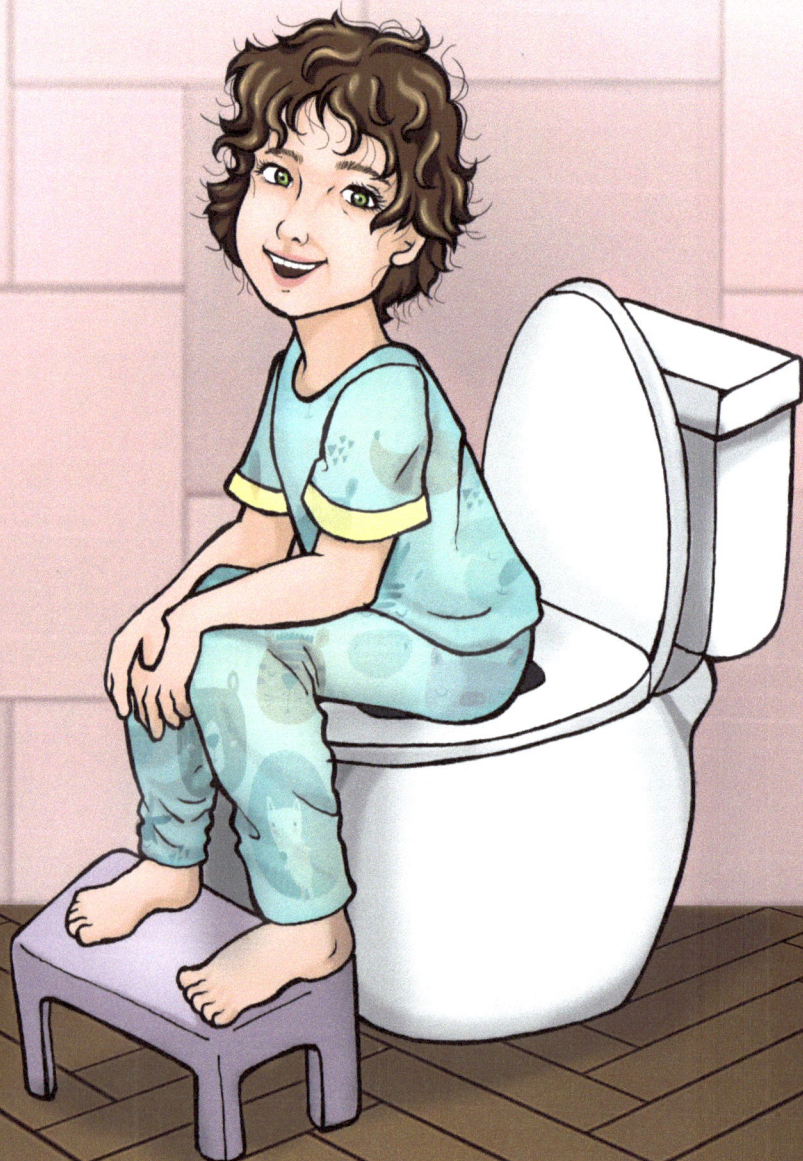

Q is for Quench.

I drink plenty of water to quench my thirst and keep my poops from drying out inside of me. I need to drink half an ounce of water for every pound that I weigh. For example, I weigh 60 lbs, so I need to drink 30 oz of water a day--more if I exercise a lot. My pee should be light yellow. I drink more if it turns darker yellow or has a strong odor.

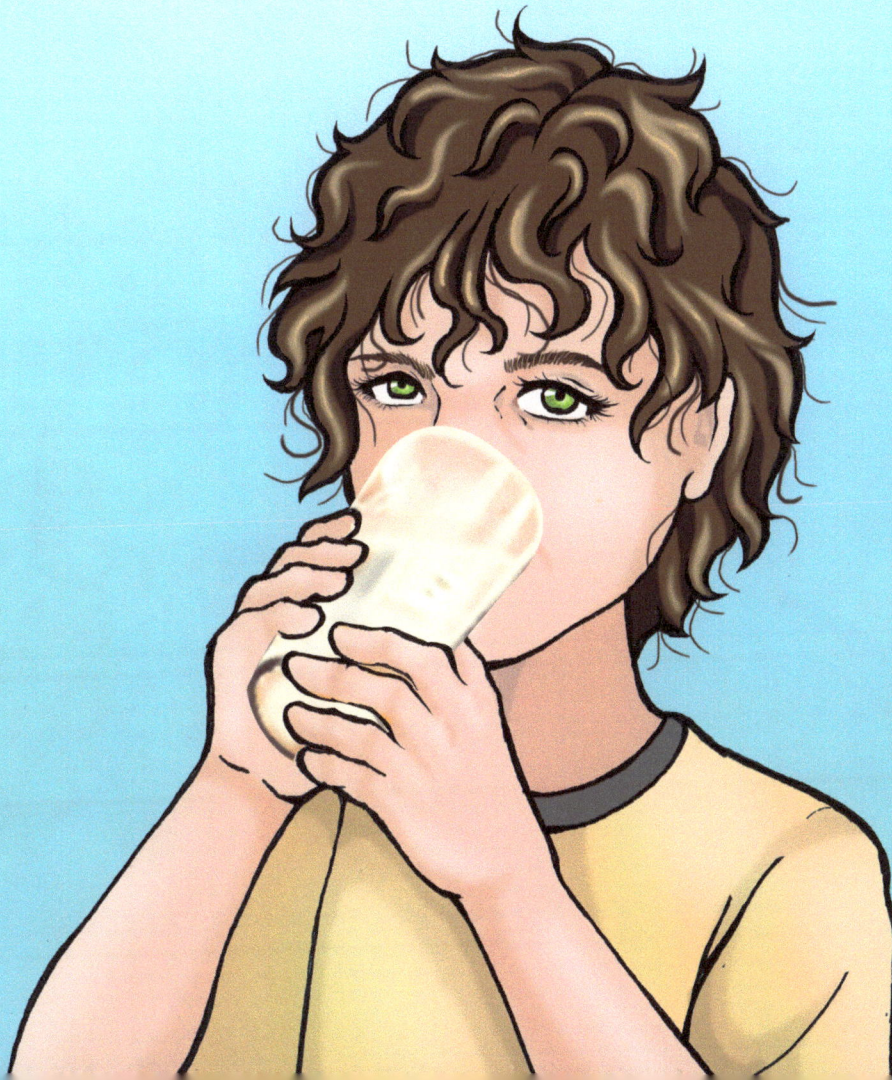

R is for Real.

I have learned the importance of eating real food. Fiber is essential to keeping my poop going through me. I need to eat more food that looks like it did in nature, like fruits and vegetables. I try to eat a rainbow of colors in my food. I need to avoid food made in factories and put in boxes and packages. Those foods make it more likely for me to get constipated again.

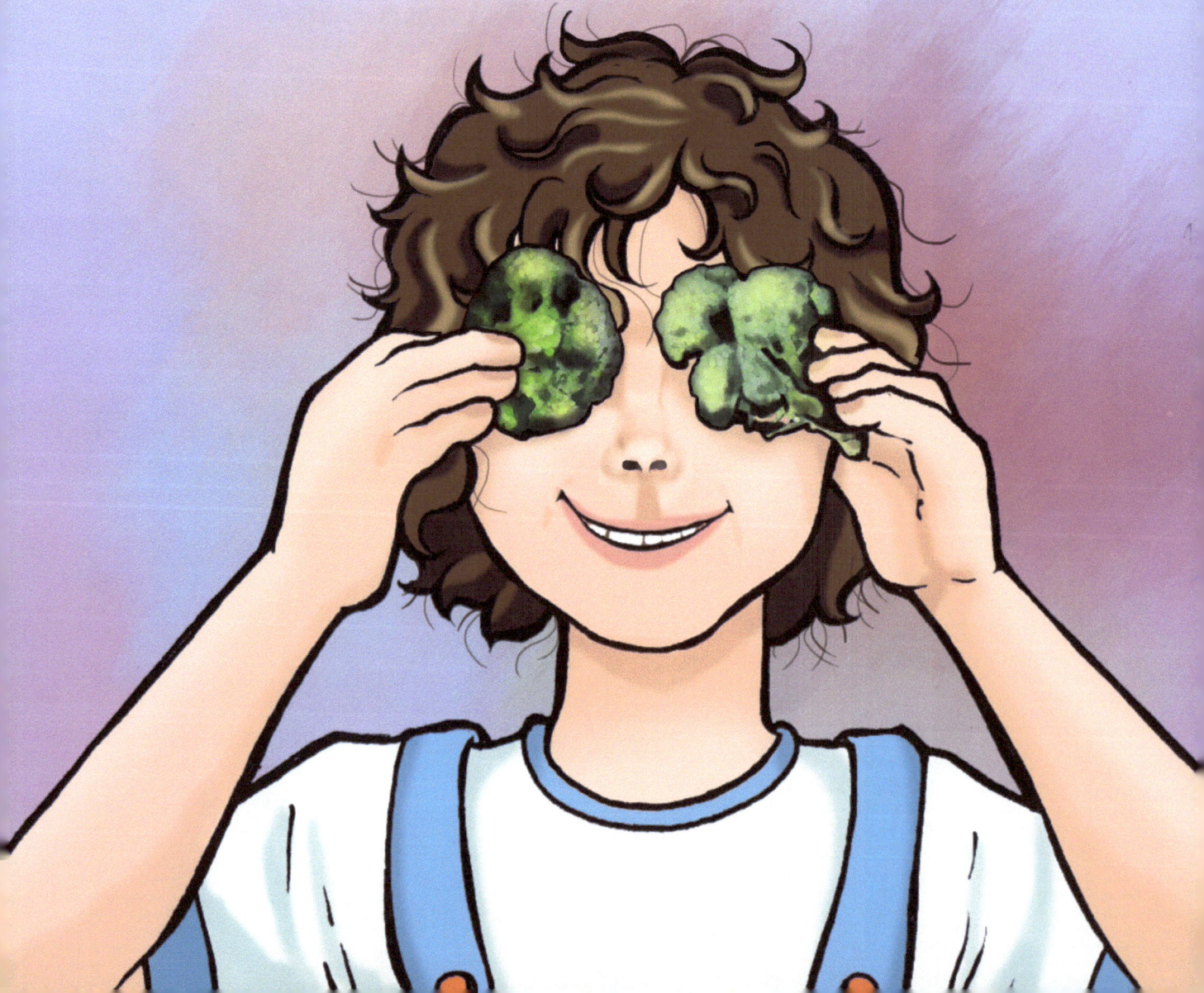

S is for Sitting.
Sitting all the time is not good for me.
Exercise helps poop pass through my body
more quickly. I wait at least an hour after eating
a meal to exercise. Mom helps me get an hour
of exercise every day. What a big difference
that has made.

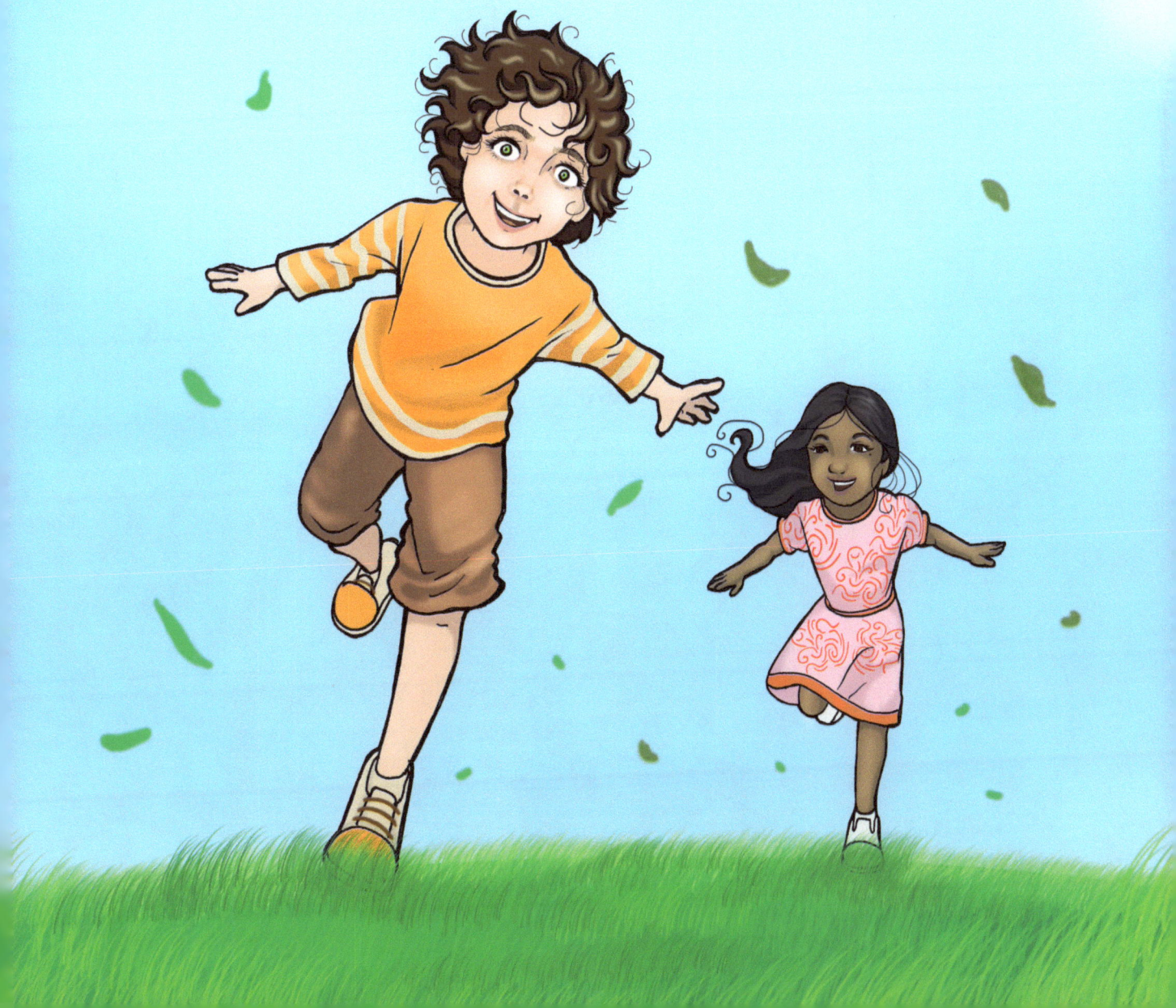

T is for Therapist.
My Dad takes me to see a therapist.
She is teaching me exercises to strengthen
the muscles that control my poop and pee,
called the pelvic floor muscles. I learned
to squeeze them light, medium, and hard.
I can now relax them, too. I learned how to
control a pee or poop urge until I can get
to the bathroom. Terrific!

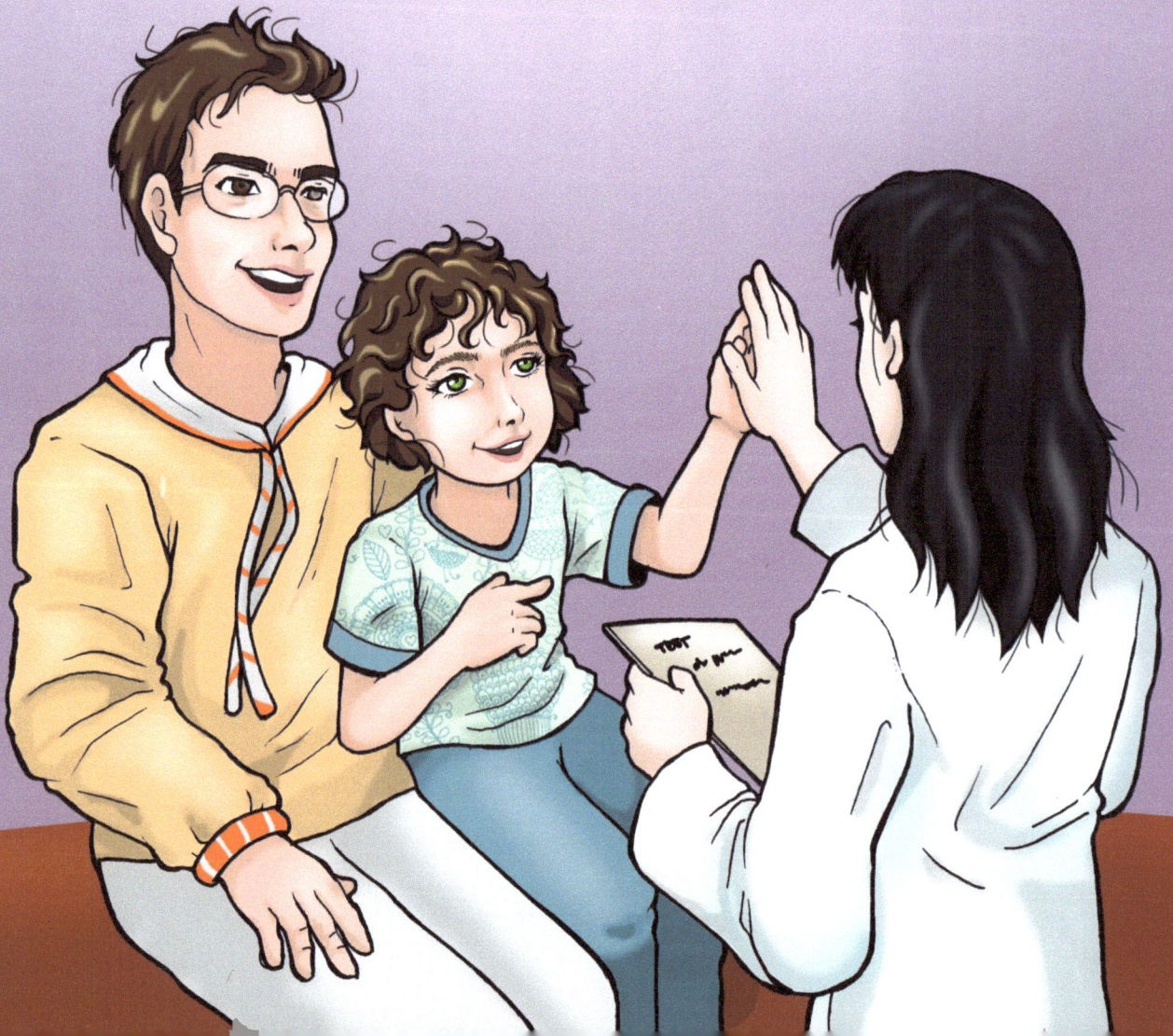

U is for Using an incentive chart.
Seeing my progress using the chart is awesome!
I get to choose my reward. Who knew pooping
and peeing could be so much fun!

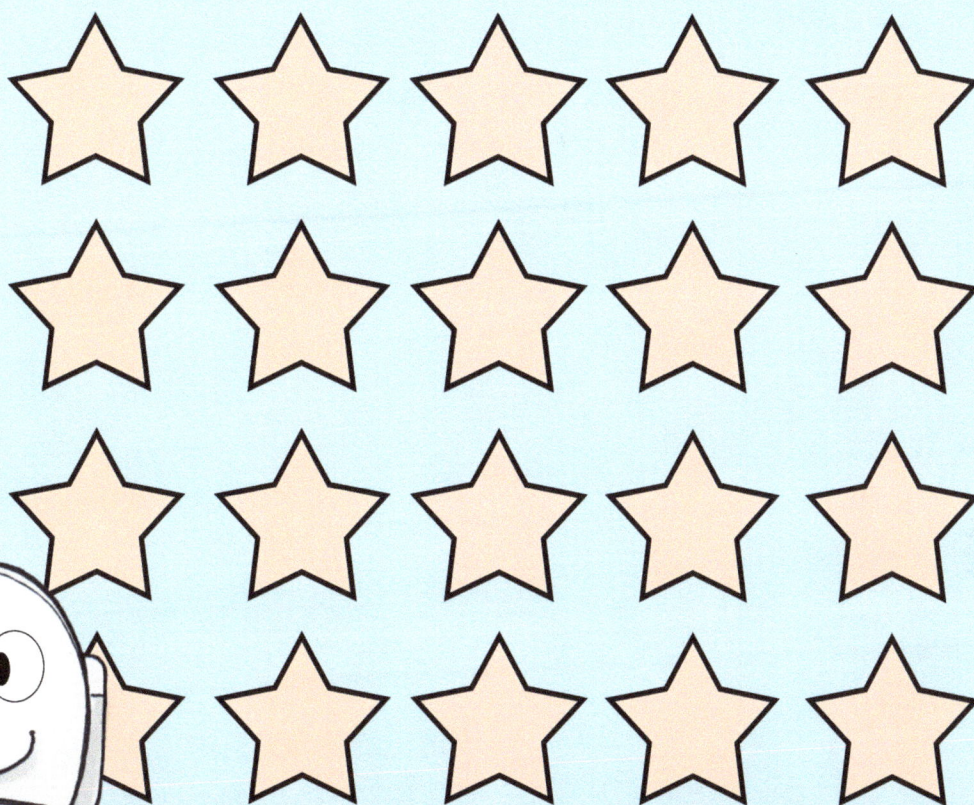

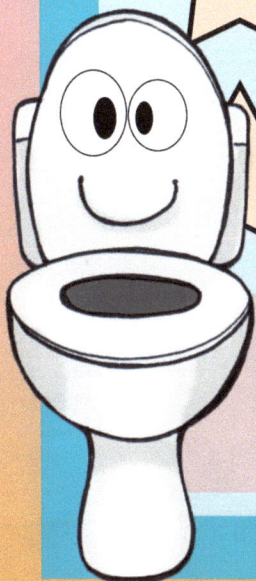

Potty Chart

V is for Very.
I am very happy this was taken care of when I was younger. Unfortunately, some people hide this problem. It can stay with them into their teens. Many adults still have problems from not handling this when they were younger.

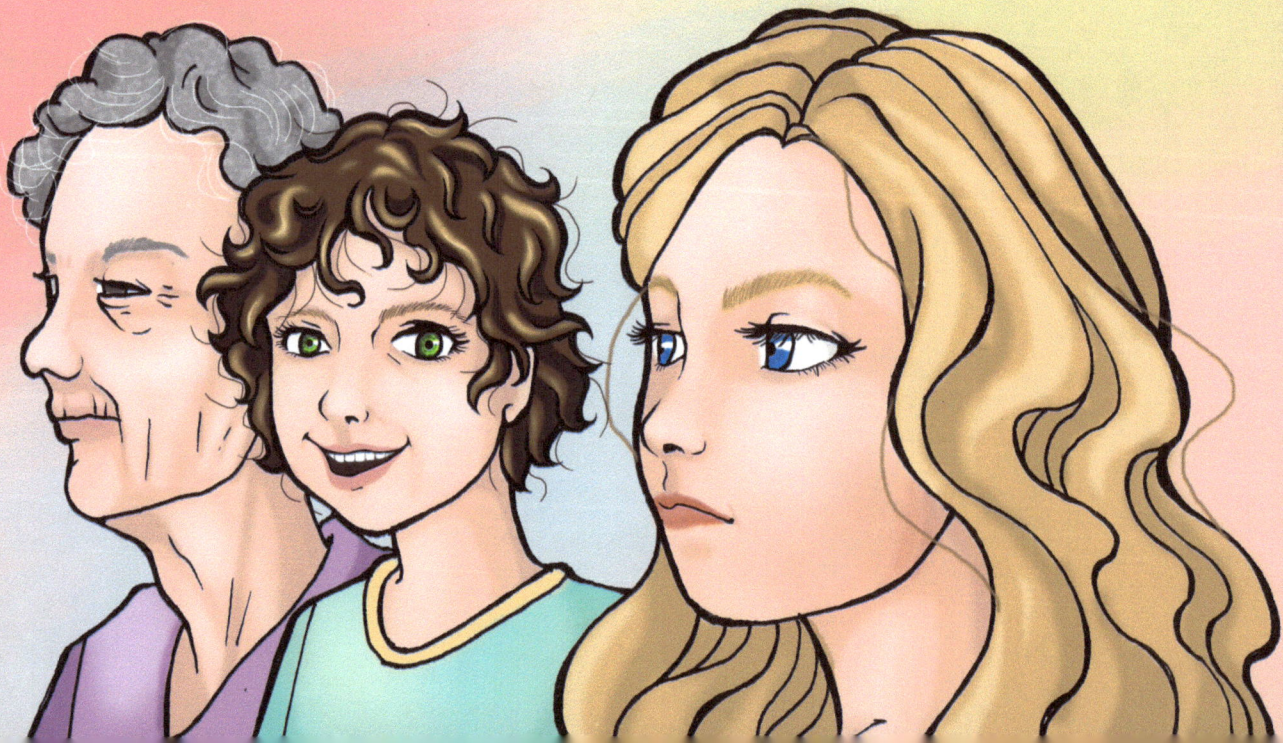

W is for What!?!!

Dad had this problem too when he was my age!?!!
Parents who have poop or pee accidents are more
likely to have children who have poop and pee
accidents. No wonder Dad understood
what I was going through.

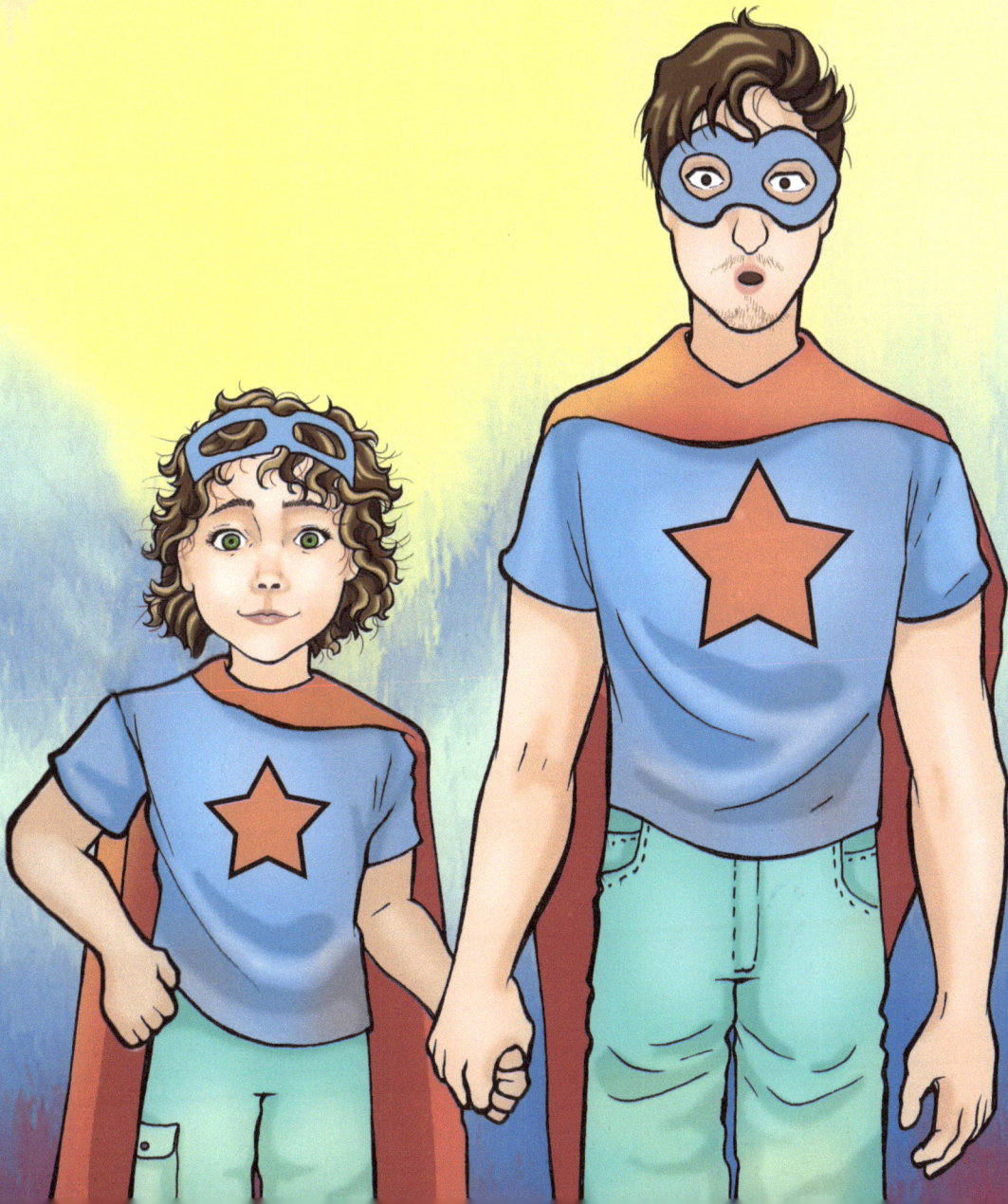

X is for eXcited.
I am excited this problem is getting
under control. How cool is it to talk about
this openly without getting so embarrassed?
I just have to stay focused on the program.

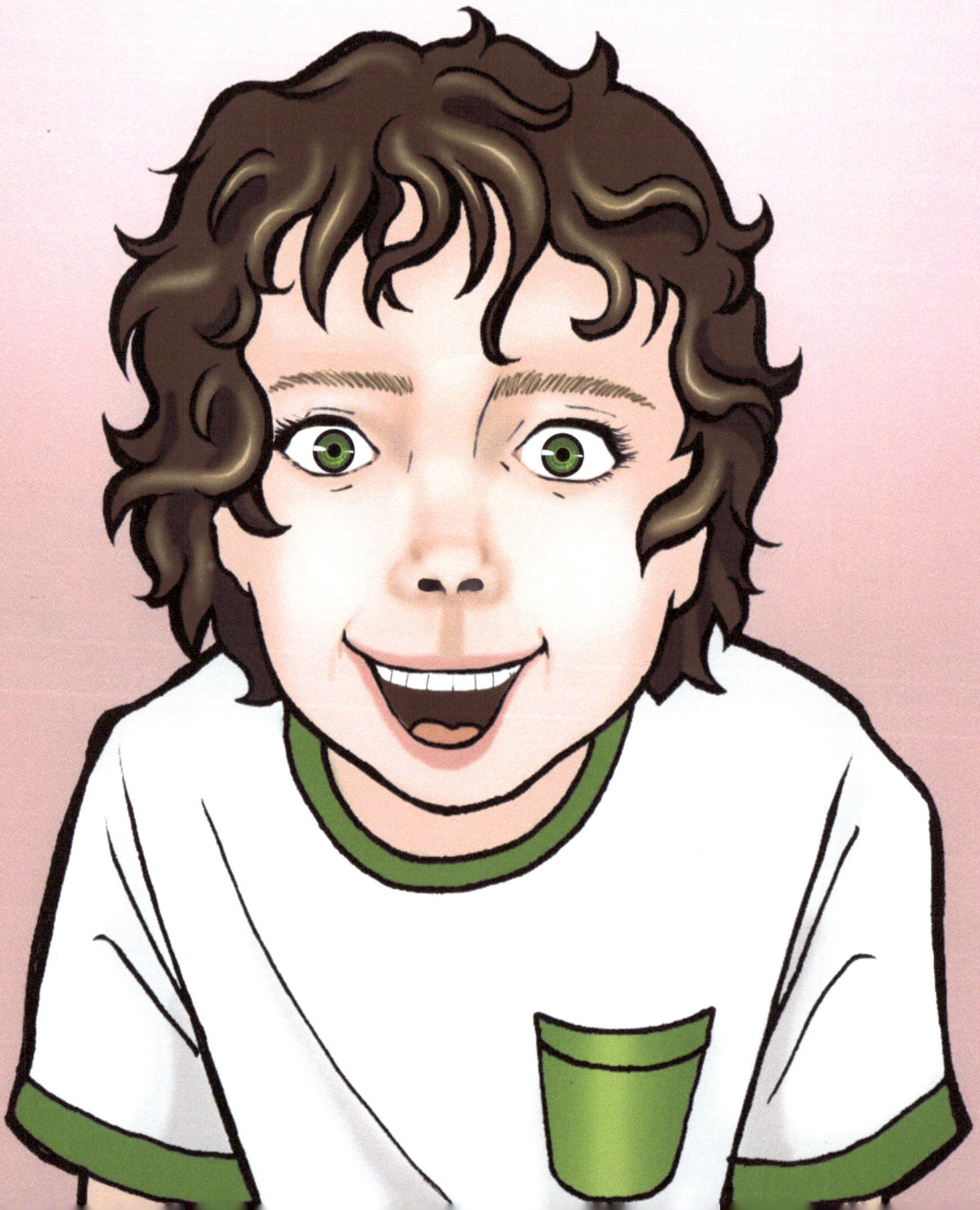

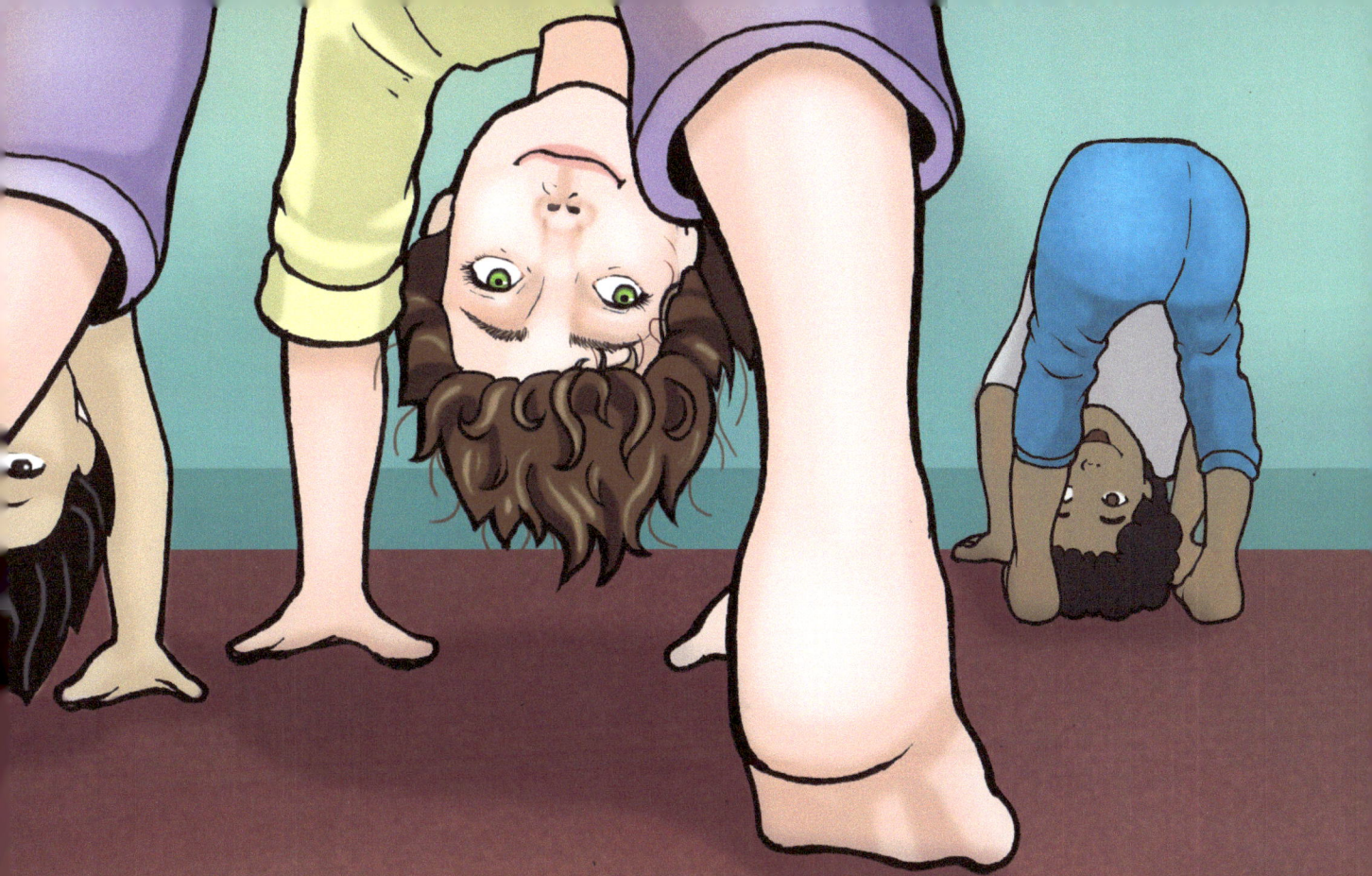

Y is for You.

Now that you know about poop and pee accidents, I hope we can be friends. I am thrilled that you understand now that it wasn't my fault. Hopefully, most of my problems are behind us now.

Z is for Zipped.
Now that I've got that problem zipped up,
let's go play!

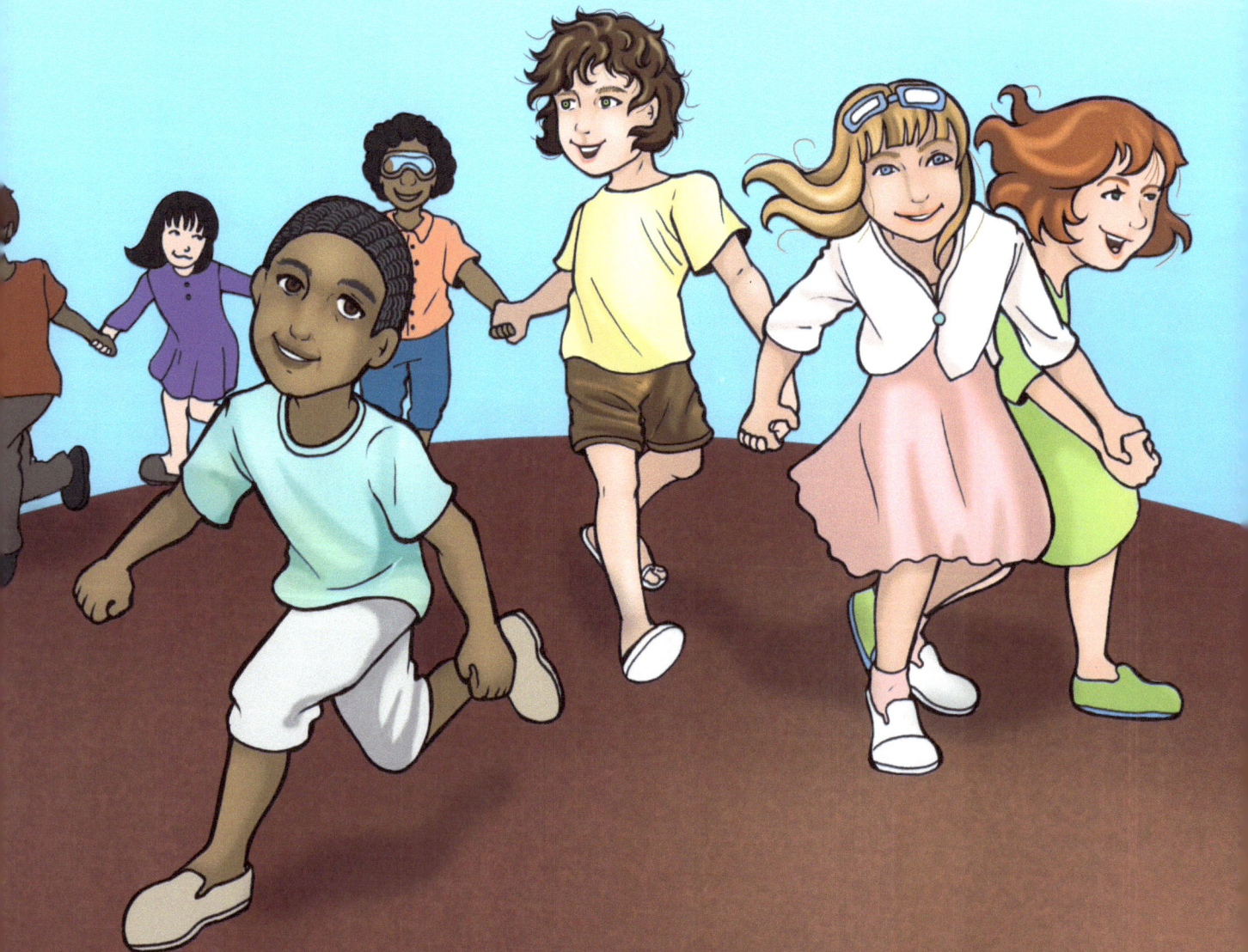

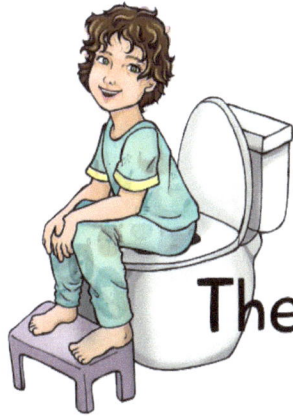

The End.

3-Step Action Plan

1. Go see a pediatric urologist.

2. Consult with a Pediatric physical therapist who specializes in encopresis and/or enuresis.

3. Diligently follow the program.

Other offerings by the author:

A is for Autism: A Child's View

D is for Down Syndrome: A Child's View

C is For Cerebral Palsy: A Child's View

A is for ADHD: A Child's View

A is for Anxiety: A Child's View

Pediatric Physical Therapy Strengthening Exercises for the Hips

Pediatric Physical Therapy Strengthening Exercises for the Knees

Pediatric Physical Therapy Strengthening Exercises for the Ankles

YouTube Channel:
Pediatric Physical Therapy Exercises

Facebook page:
Pediatric Physical Therapy Exercises

Instagram page:
Pediatric PT Exercises

Blog:
www.pediatricPTexercises.com

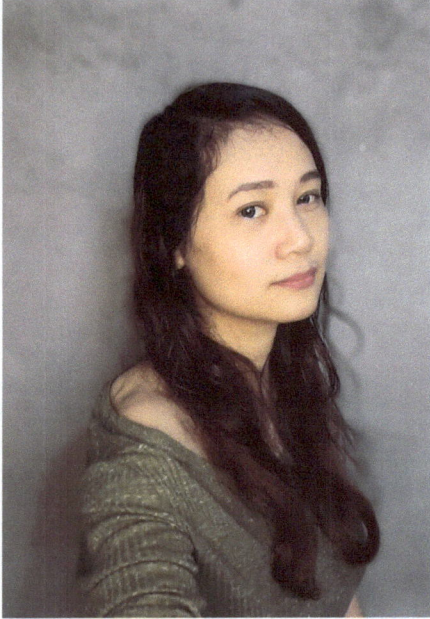

Ikos Ronzkie is an international comic strip artist, book illustrator, and graphic designer. She creates fantastical images for advertisements, campaigns, comic books, character designs, book designs, and book covers.

She has over 16 years of experience as an illustrator, serving both domestic and foreign clients.

She illustrated this author's previous books, *A is for Autism, D is for Down Syndrome, C is for Cerebral Palsy, A is for Attention Deficit Hyperactivity Disorder,* and *A is for Anxiety.* She is also the illustrator for books, including *My Daddy's Hat, Pirate Sam, There's a Mermaid in my Bathtub, What's Wrong with Grandma?, My Tooth Fairy,* and *Willie Nilly Adventures.*

She created *Bayan ng Biyahero comics* for a Local Newspaper and *Estudyante Blues comics* for the Living News and Good Education Magazine. Independently, she writes and produces her own comics.

She founded MINT (*Mama, Ilaw Ng Tahanan*), a group for Filipina Moms to meet people, make friends, find support, explore your interests or even grow a business.

She also co-founded, with her husband, *Ru's Nest.* It is a page that they describe as their online love letter to their son, Ru. Their contents focus on their love for Ru and as they explore his fleeting interests as a child. They share with their son the experience of experimenting with things that they, as a couple, are passionate about.

She is the co-founder of *Allawig Studio,* which strives to promote and explore Philippine culture with visual arts. Their creations are dedicated to work inspired by Philippine history, myths, and legends.

She recently co-founded *ScarAbs,* with her husband, an art studio for their commercial illustrations that focuses on mythical creatures from various cultures.

She recently co-founded *Yellow Lobster,* with her husband, an art studio that caters for kids and kids at heart as they produce cute and whimsical illustrations.

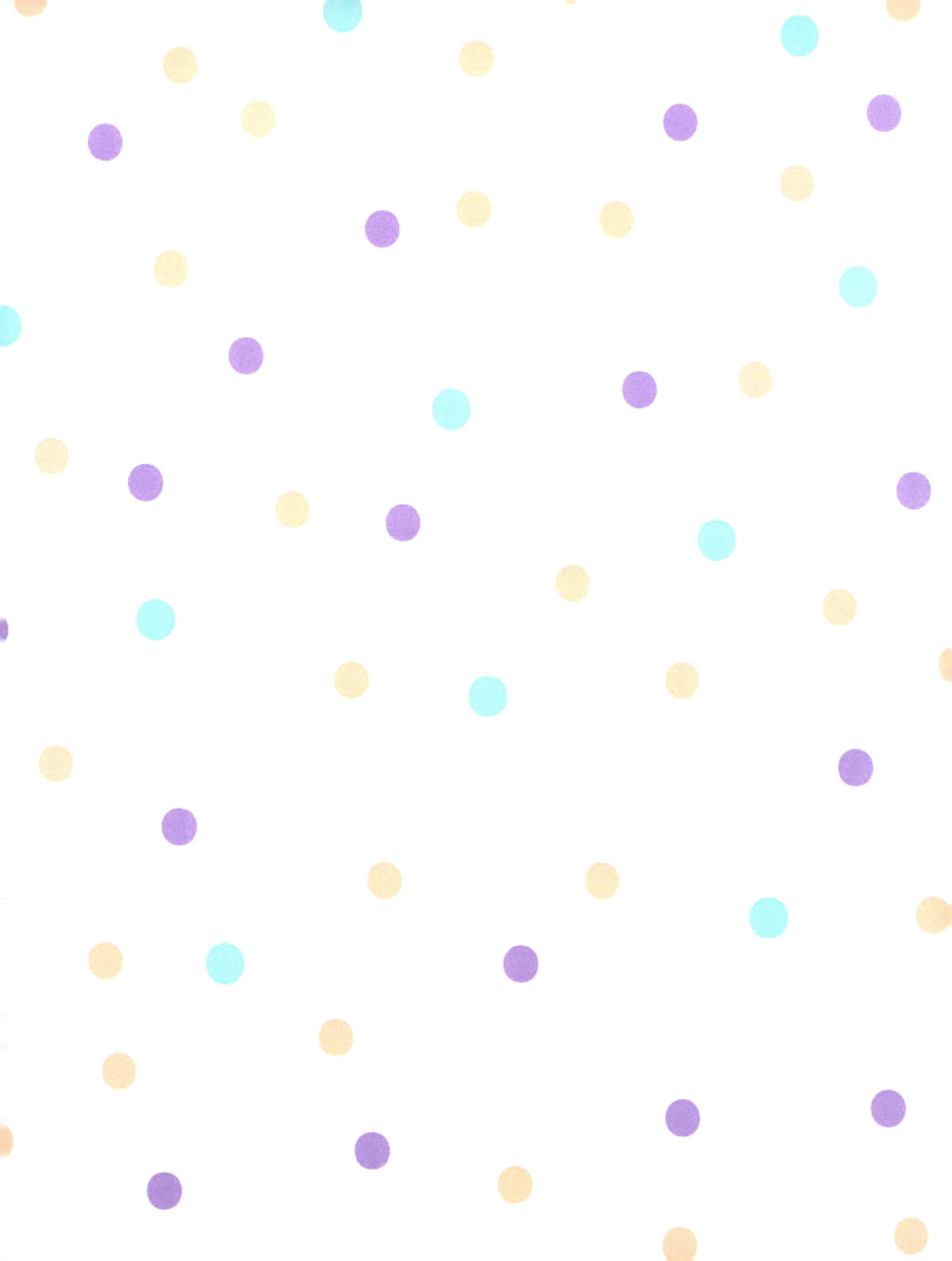

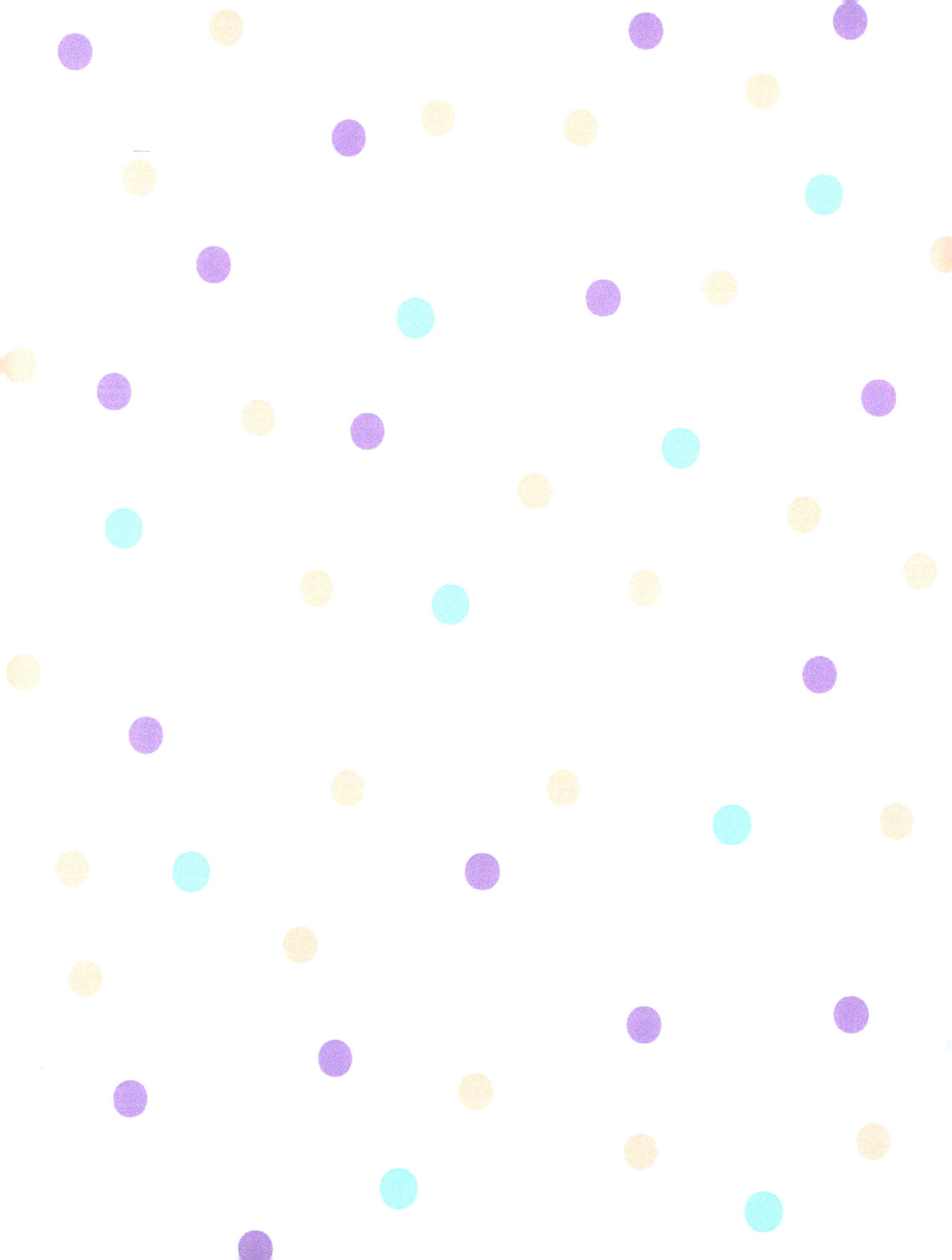

www.ingramcontent.com/pod-product-compliance
Lightning Source LLC
Chambersburg PA
CBHW060834270326
41933CB00002B/80